Gudrun Bornhöft

HAPPINESS – OF THE SOUL AND OF SWINE

A Sounder of Life's Wisdom

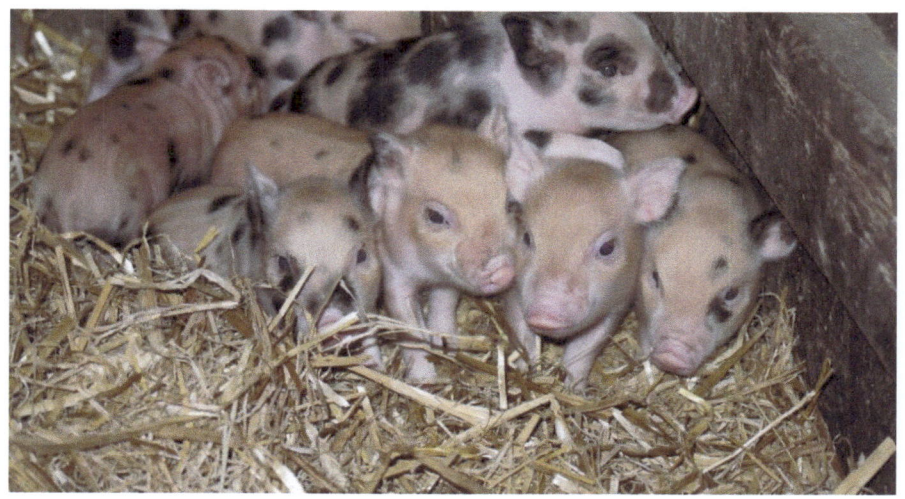

(NI)

Translated by Steffi Cook and Sonja Ahrens (and revised by James Kershaw)

Books on Demand GmbH, Norderstedt, 2016

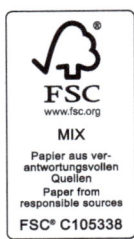

Happiness – of the Soul and of Swine

© 2016 Gudrun Bornhöft: gudrun.bornhoeft@online.de

Photos by Hansjörg Bornhöft © 2012-2014

Translated by Steffi Cook and Sonja Ahrens (and revised by James Kershaw)

Produced and published by:
BoD - Books on Demand, Norderstedt
ISBN 9783743119178

Gudrun Bornhöft

HAPPINESS – OF THE SOUL AND OF SWINE

A Sounder of Life's Wisdom

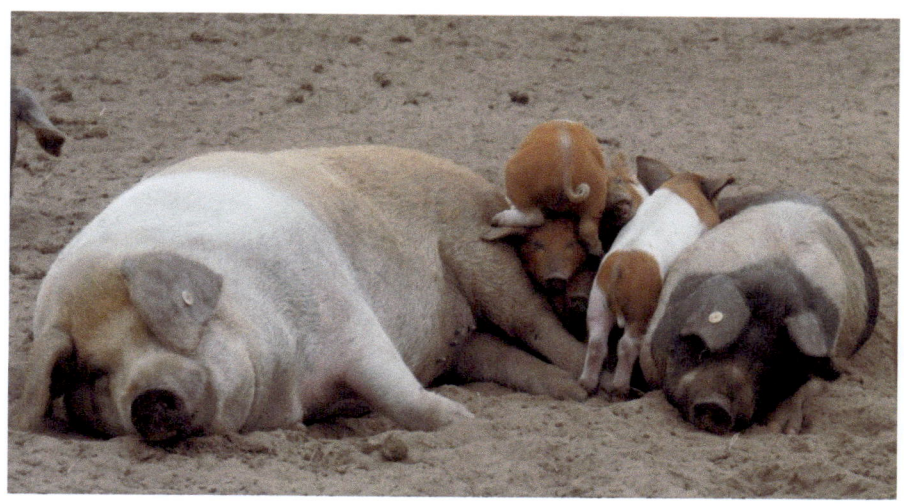

(NF)

Translated by Steffi Cook and Sonja Ahrens (and revised by James Kershaw)

For my dear husband Hansjörg who makes each day a joyful one for me

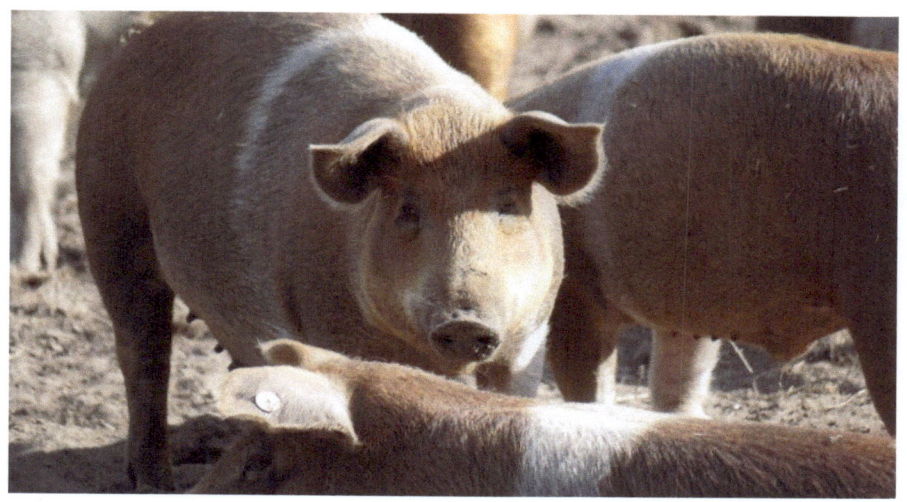

(NF)

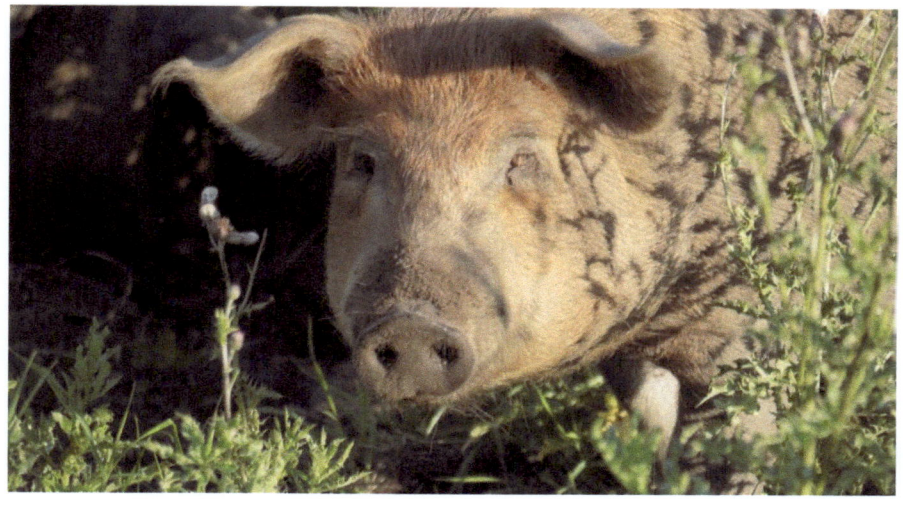

(NF)

Introductory thoughts

Why a book about happiness, the soul and pigs? Purely to create joy! Using pigs? **Of course!** Who can resist the charm of these inquisitive creatures? It is remarkable how expressive, how full of life pigs can be when we respect them as sensitive creatures rather than abuse them as common goods; this applies to almost anything we approach full of loving respect.

And to prepare the way for some spirituality to enter our lives. – Using pigs? Let's give it a go.
Spirituality need not be esoteric or synonymous with religion, although there is room for both in a comprehensive spirituality. It can also include the conviction that a spirituality by itself does not exist– everything can be understood ‚in some way or another' as an emergence from material systems.
Regardless of our attitude to spirituality, our lives are more spiritual than we know.
When we see this symbol

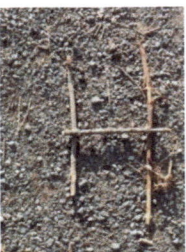

we may assume it *is* the letter ‚h'. Children of Kindergarten age see two straight sticks and another one across, Russians may see it as the letter ‚n'. It is our idea more than the sensual perception that determines what it really *is*. At the same time it is noteworthy that we are capable of viewing something from another's perspective and to identify with it (as long as it seems plausible). Generally speaking: reality *is* indeed imagination.
I am convinced that there is a separate universal spirit, distinct from our human spirit, that it is infinite, eternal and dynamic and that it has a consciousness all of its own. One can regard this spirit as God, or choose

to view it as something else. An alternative way of looking at this would be to imagine a meaningful space (*Bedeutungsraum*). Everything is represented in this space as spiritual models – as thoughts of the universal spirit. These models interact with their corresponding physical counterparts according to their respective innate laws (e.g. using resonance). The interaction of an individual spiritual mode with a human body allows human consciousness as we know it to evolve as an emergent ‚product' or epiphenomenon. This consciousness affects both system components resulting in a modified spiritual mode, which after death can join another physical being.

In life we experience the harmonious resonance of the components of both systems as joy: the physical system with its components: constitution, organs and actions; the spiritual with character, awareness, and aspiration. The choice of spiritual modes that resonate with us and that we wish to strengthen is for the individual to decide; a choice representing both free will and accountability.

There are many photos of pigs and piglets in this book. We visited them mainly at these four locations (abbreviations of locations in brackets next to the pictures):

- (LRO): Farm Animal Park Lelkendorf, Rostock area
- (RD): Farm Animal Park Arche Warder, Rendsburg-Eckernförde area
- (NI): Brand-Aue (for minipigs) in Rodewald, later Pennigsehl, both Nienburg/Weser area
- (NF): Hockmannshof in Humptrup (the Husum Red Pied or ‚Danish Protest Pig'), North Frisia

Pigs and Notes

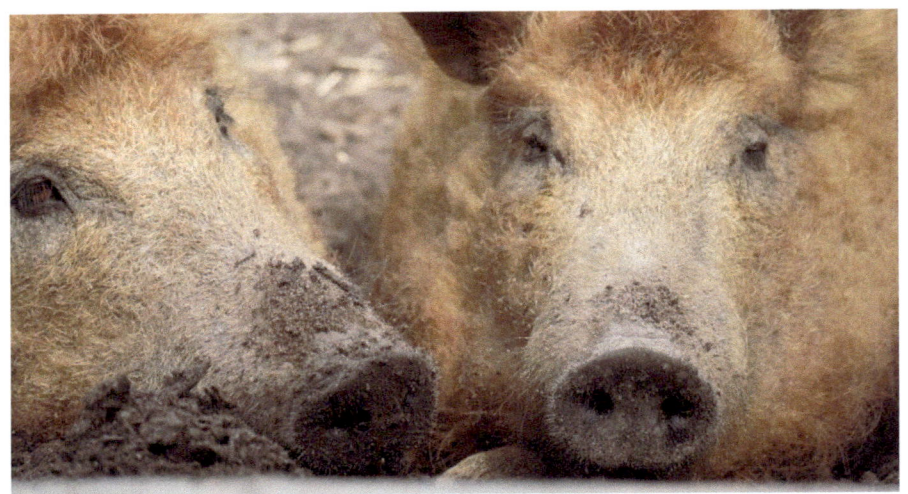

(RD)

" "If we learn to feel joy we will unlearn how to hurt others." [Nietzsche]
(" „All men will be brothers dwelling under the safety of your wings.")

("Alle Menschen werden Brüder, wo dein sanfter Flügel weilt" [Schiller])

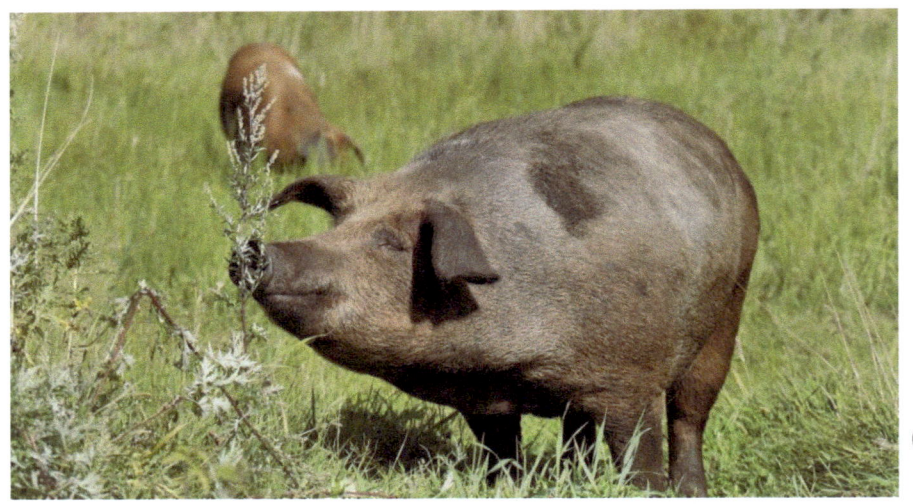

(NF)

" I believe that the purpose of life is to be happy."[Tenzin Gyatso, 14. Dalai Lama in: http://www.dalailama.com/messages/compassion]

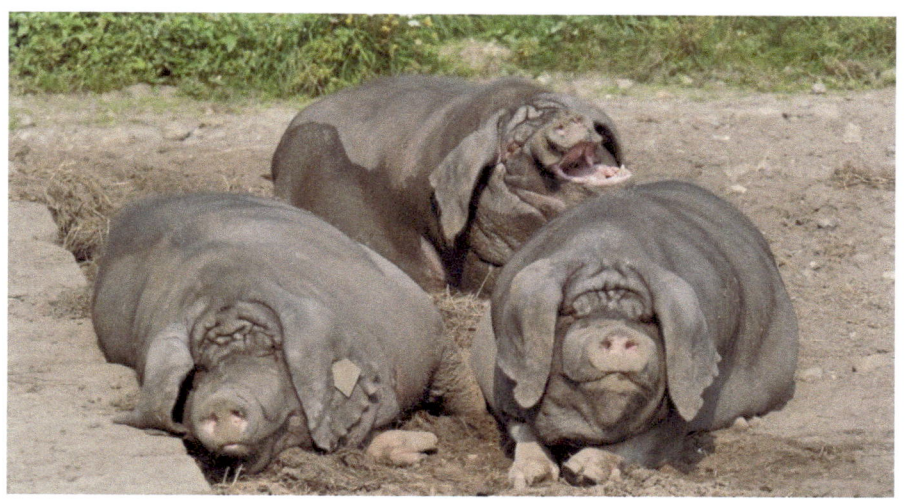 (RD)

"Society's aim is universal happiness." [Article 1 of the French Constitution of 1793 which did not come into force]

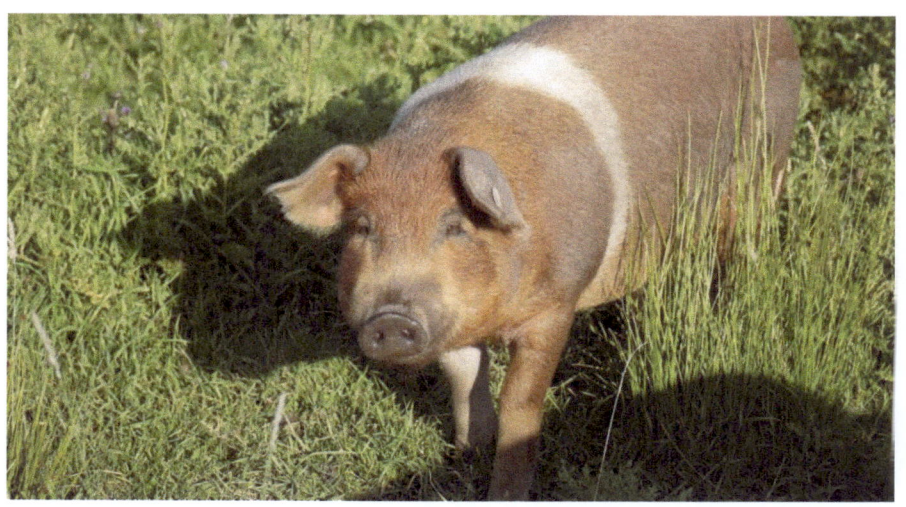 (NF)

To strive for your own and others' happiness is a noble aim.

Für sich und Andere nach Glück sehr viel
zu streben ist ein edles Ziel.

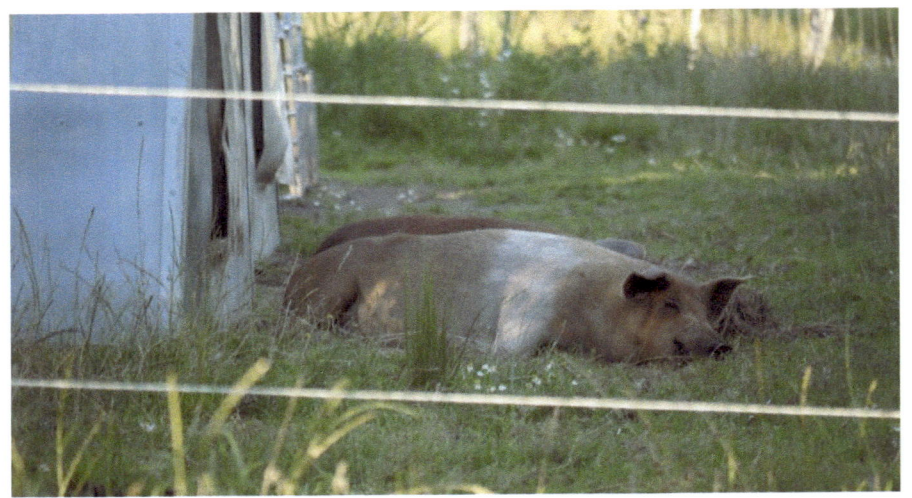 (NF)

Not to be hungry, not to be cold – and to feel joy.

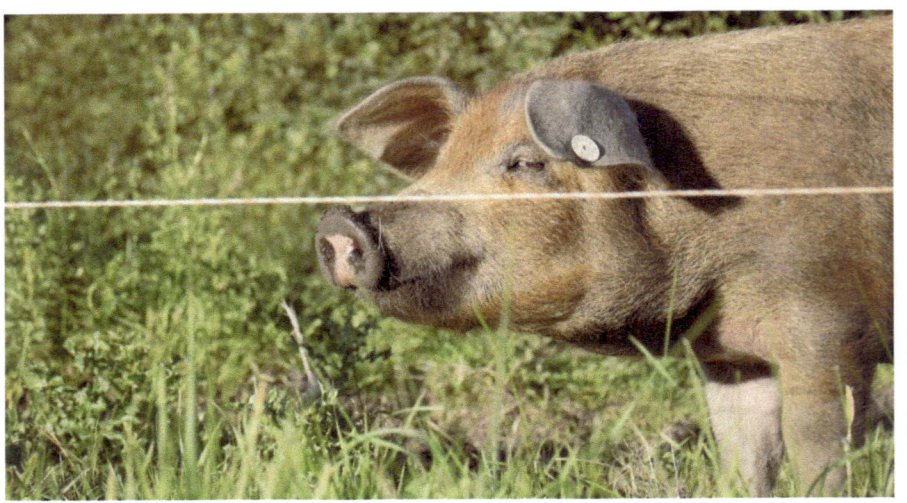 (NF)

Any money that is not transformed into joy of living amounts to merely numbers on paper.
" Modesty equals freedom." [José Mujica]

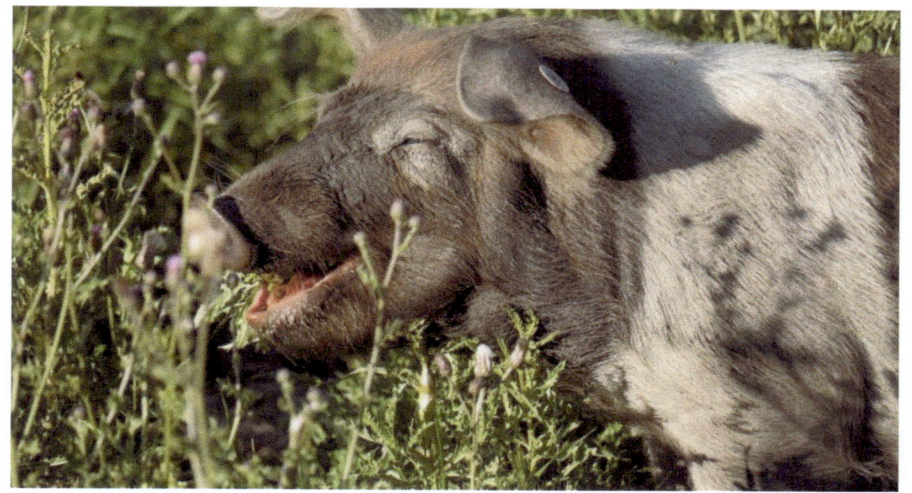

True happiness is being and doing, not possessions or results.

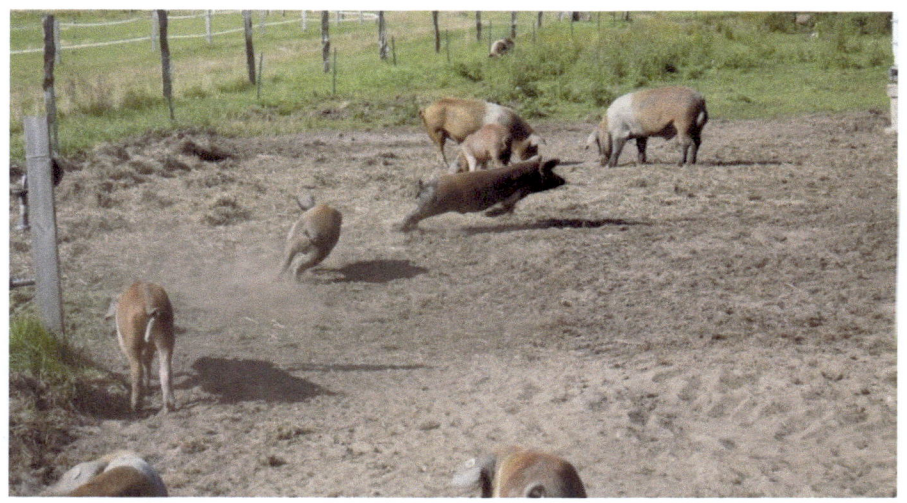

Each knock life deals us can be healed by joy.

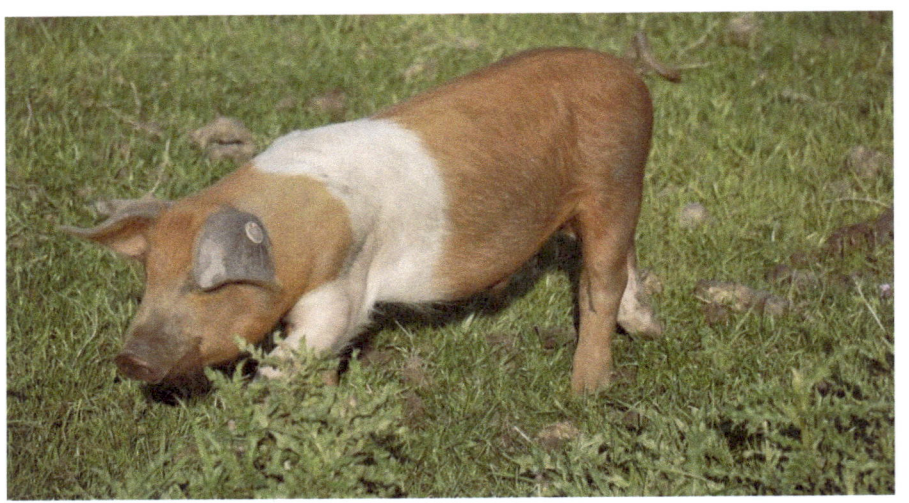

(NF)

To open yourself to spirituality, can be a life led quite happily. But to close, can lead to life morose.	*Zu öffnen sich der Geistigkeit, Führt einen zur Glückseligkeit; Sich aber zu verschließen, Kann's Leben sehr verdrießen.*

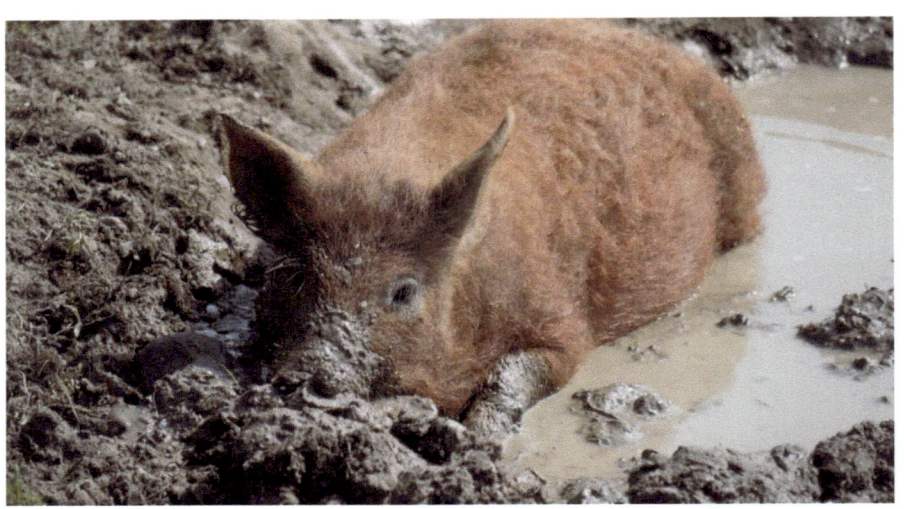

(RD)

The same applies in death: open yourself for heaven with your last breath; let not your soul close in fear, or forever shed in hell your tear.	*Im Tod ist's dann genauso gleich, Sich Öffnen führt ins Himmelreich; Doch schließt die Seel' sich ängstlich ein, Erleidet sie nur Höllenpein.*

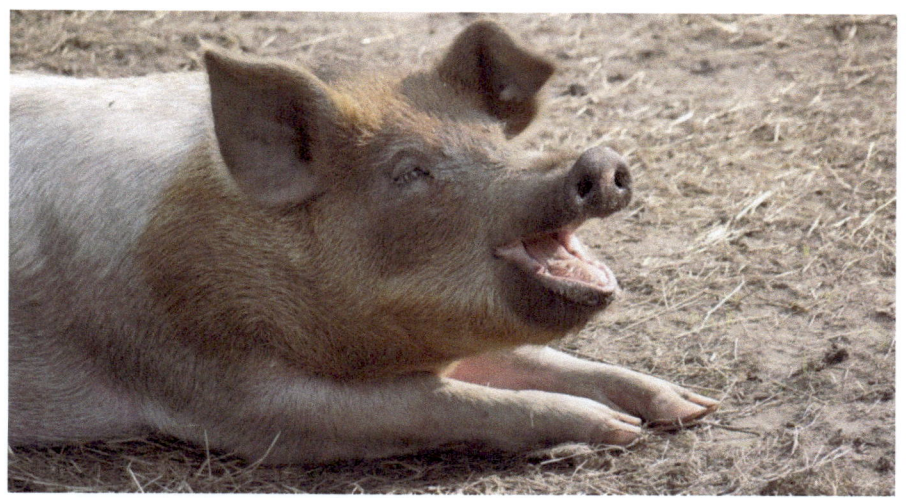
(NF)

"Death does not concern us, because as long as we exist, death is not here. And once it does come, we no longer exist." [Epicurius]
Death is stronger than any anaesthetic.

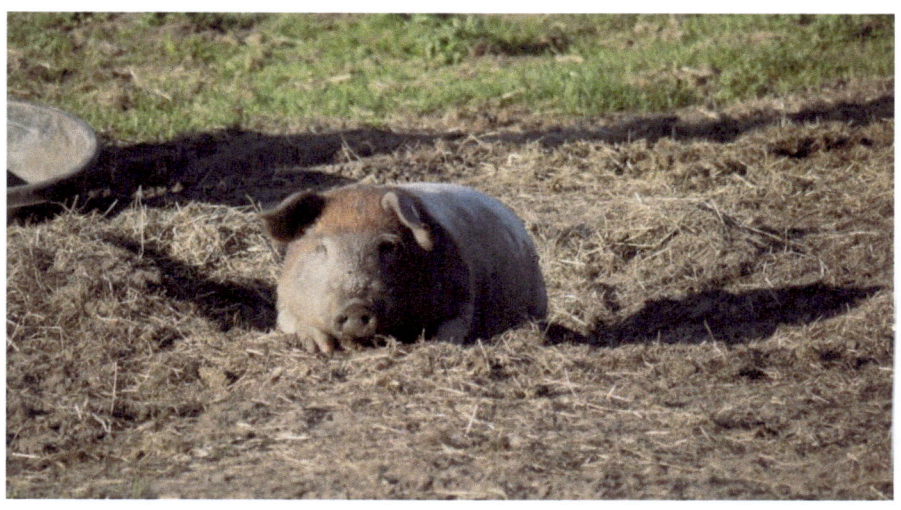
(NF)

And my soul spread	Und meine Seele spannte
Its wings out wide,	Weit ihre Flügel aus.
And flew through the peaceful countryside,	Flog durch die stillen Lande, Als flöge sie nach Haus.
as though it were going home.	[Eichendorff]

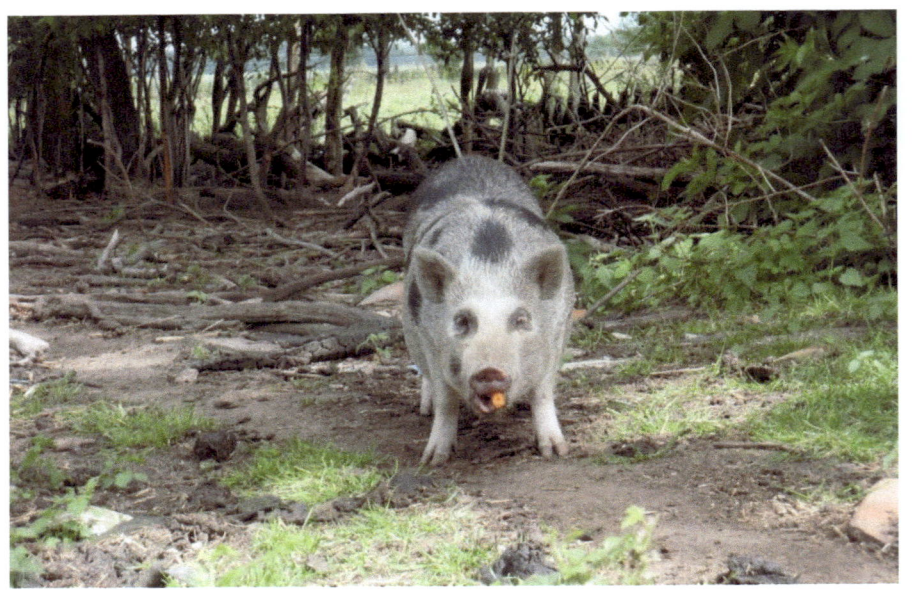
(NI)

Every thought and every decision has a spiritual effect. They weave spiritual modes which we add to our spiritual being.
Spiritual systems recognise one another.

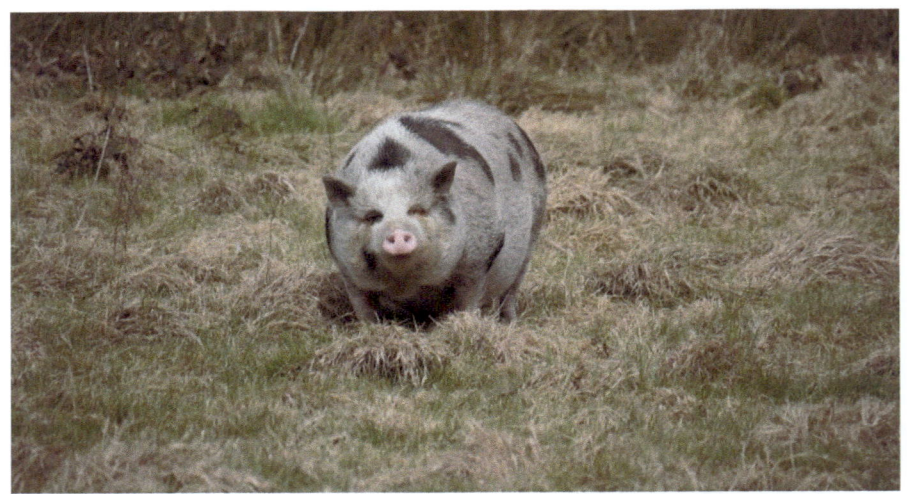
(NI)

" For what shall it profit a man, if he shall gain the whole world, and lose his own soul?" [St Mark's 8:36]

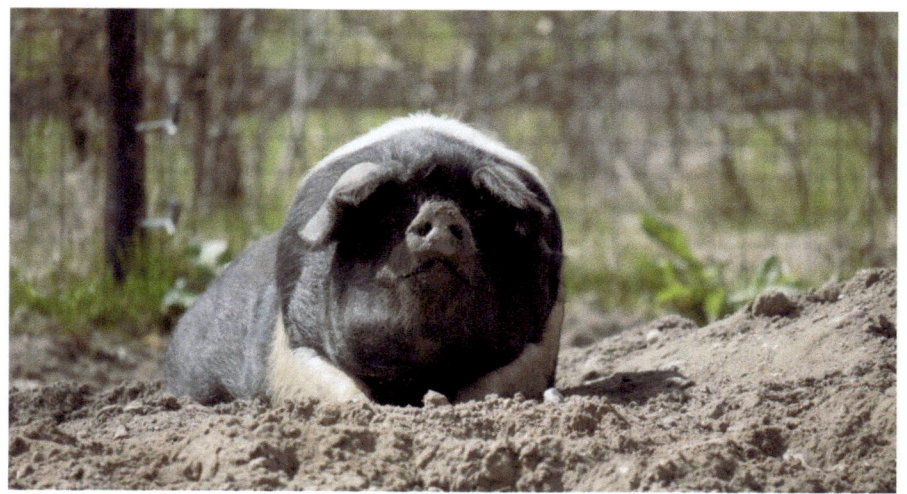

(RD)

Those who meditate in life are dealt a better hand in the after-life.

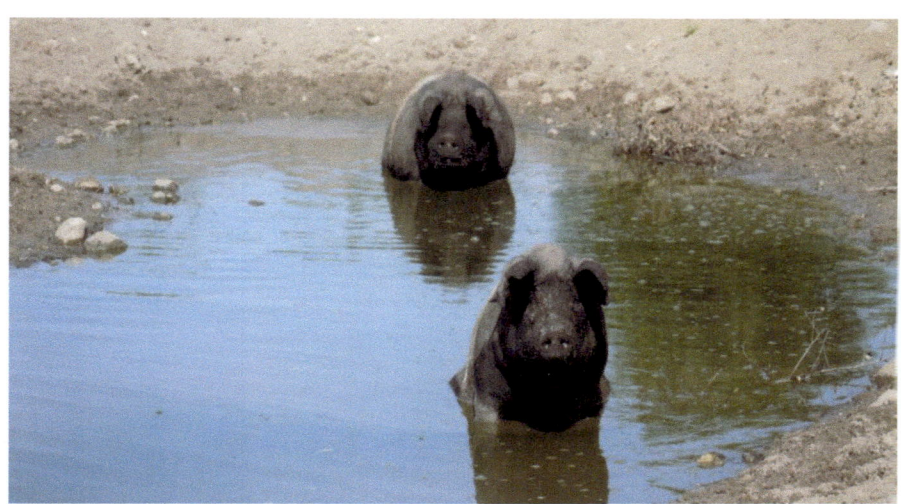

(RD)

If you do not protect your soul from evil, your spirit will be like the picture of Dorian Gray.

Hältst du die Seele nicht von Übel frei, Gleicht dein Geist dem Bild von Dorian Gray.

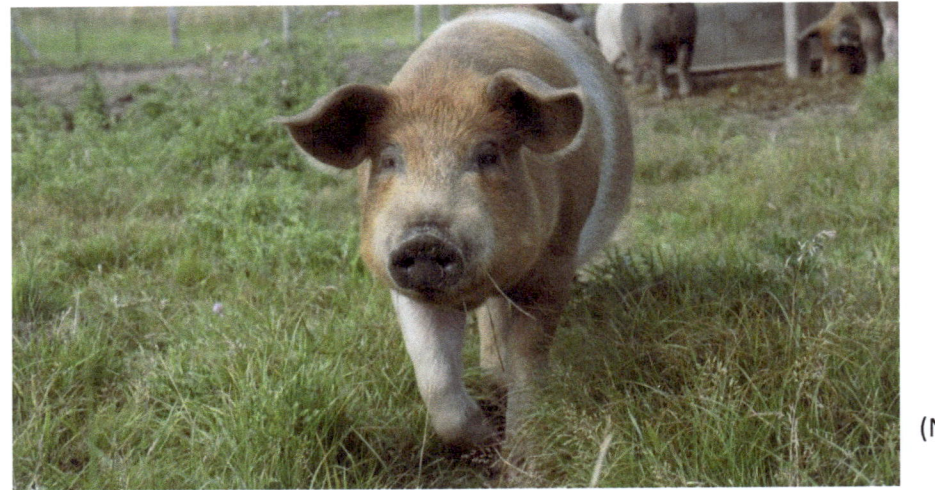

(NF)

Man determines his aspirations.

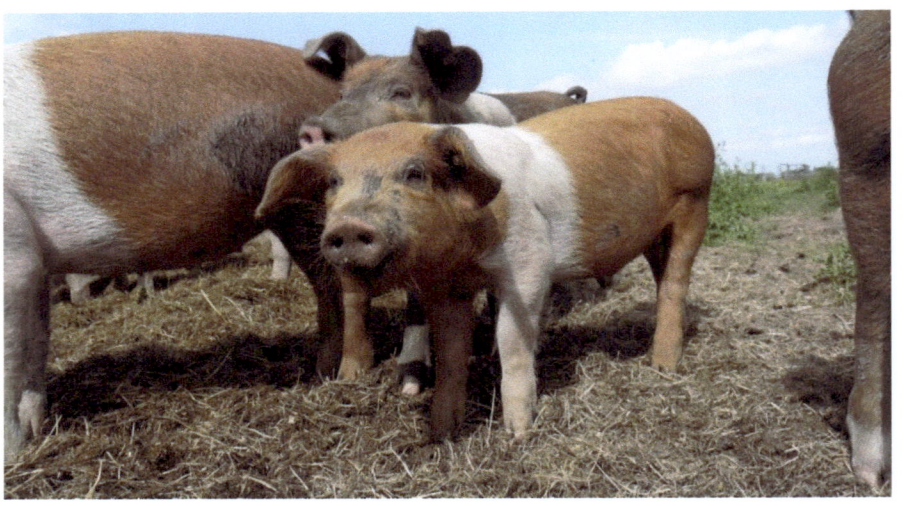

(NF)

The aim of education is to enable self determination.

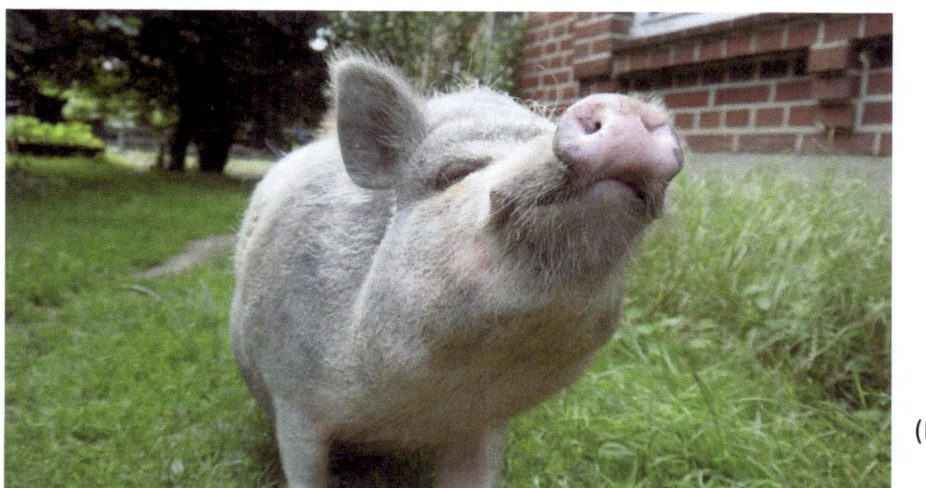

(NI)

"Sapere aude!" (Dare to know, dare to be wise. Have courage to use your own sense of reason!) [Motto from the age of enlightenment]

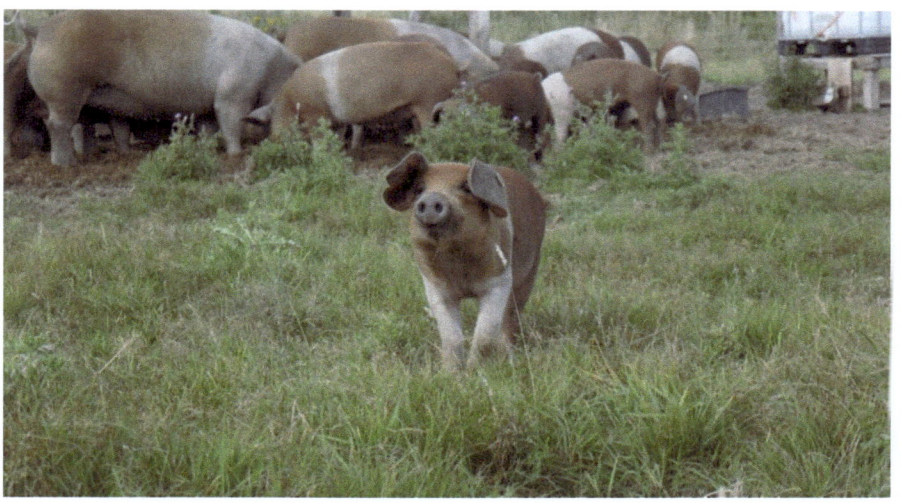

(NF)

The problem with freedom is that others could make different choices from your own. There is no obligation to act sensibly, but there is an obligation to carry the responsibility for the consequences.

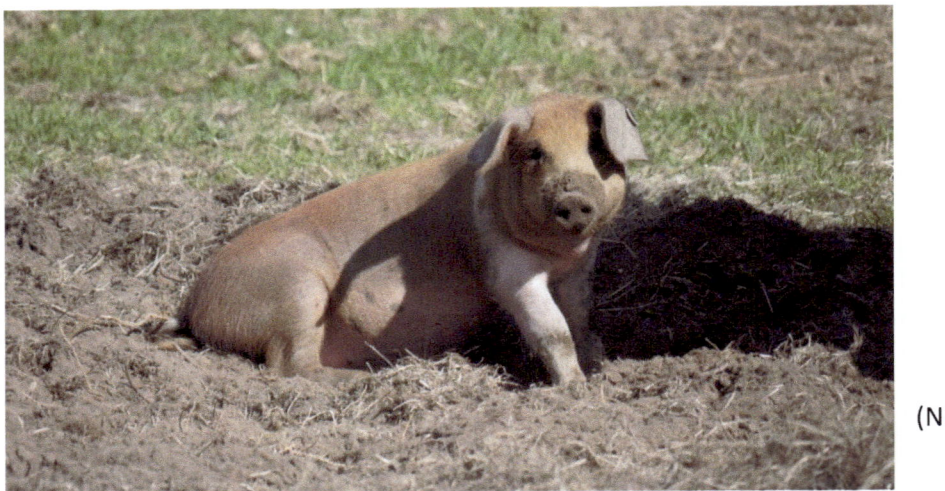
(NF)

The more I understand, the better I can decide.

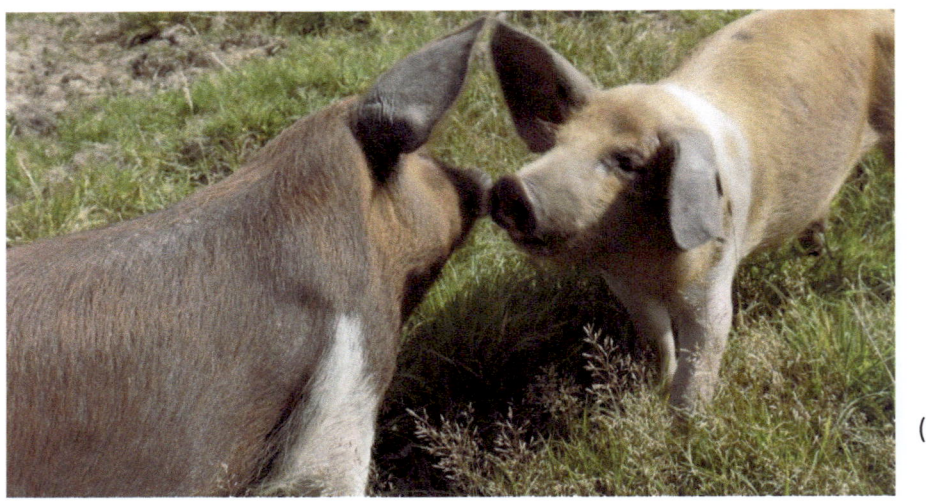
(NF)

To understand means to relate to, not agree with. To explain means to enable understanding, not to convince.

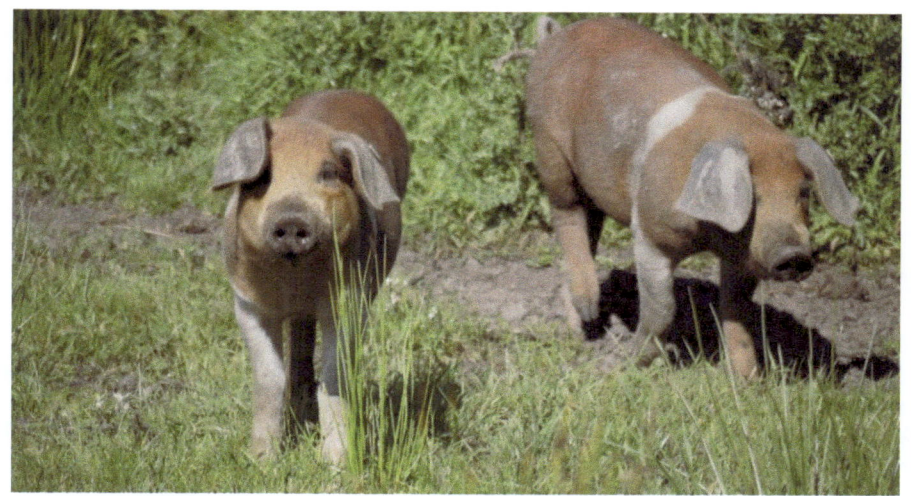
(NF)

One removes the foundation of joy if one thinks 'eliminate' rather than 'understand'. 'Restorative justice' – in contrast to 'punishment' - retains the possibility for understanding and renewed joy ("Your magics bind again, what custom has strictly parted." *Deine Zauber binden wieder, was die Mode streng geteilt."* [Schiller])
"One cannot forbid everything one does not approve of." [Thomas de Maizière]

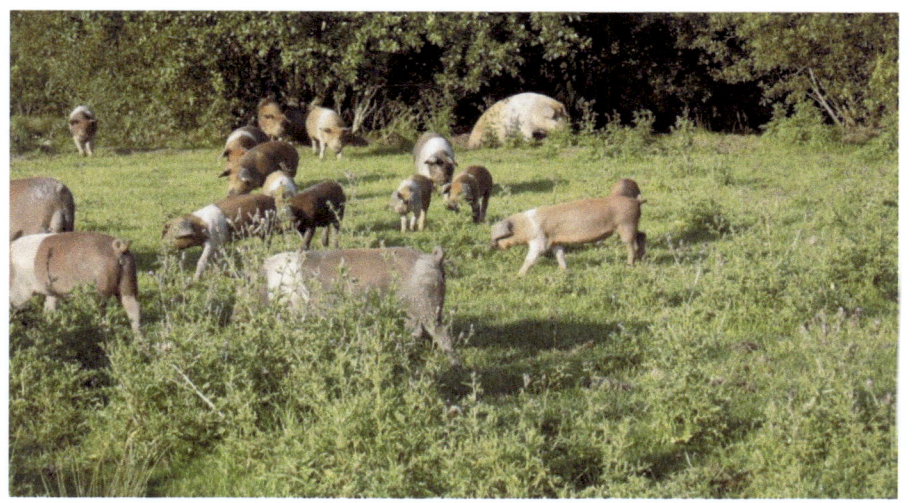
(NF)

Joy is an active movement of opening up and resonating with others. Others can only influence the conditions, e.g. they may try to reduce suffering and enable others to participate in society, which should include setting achievable goals.

The external influence on the system is the pig on the right which supports the pink one.

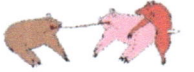 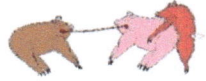

1) The system result is in line with the extent of the external influence.

2) The counter reaction prevails.

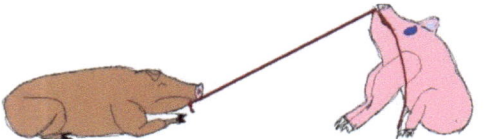

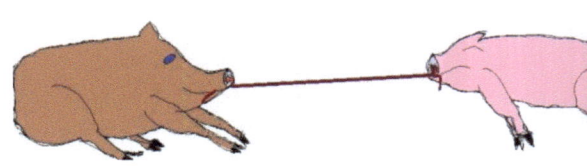

There are the laws of expansion, self organisation (with emergence), resonance, system reactions and those of more familiar subjects such as physics, biology and psychology. However, be careful not to generalise inappropriately!
Each condition which has not come about through self organisation is perceived as an external influence.

Direct external influence (refer left) and counter reaction are often easily recognisable in systems and are in part subject to mechanical laws.

Spiritual health

Man will devour much:
Contempt, anger, lovesickness.
And everyone asks, quietly horrified:
What will this lead to in the end? But see!
Only goodness and upliftedness.
Man has such an amazing digestive system

[after Eugen Roth]

Seelische Gesundheit

Ein Mensch frisst viel in sich hinein:
Missachtung, Ärger, Liebespein.
Und jeder fragt mit stillem Graus:
Was kommt da wohl einmal heraus?
Doch sieh! Nur Güte und Erbauung.
Der Mensch hat prächtige Verdauung.

[Eugen Roth]

If the laws are known, many results can be explained, but may be difficult to predict.

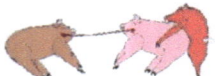 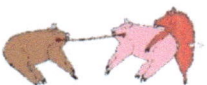

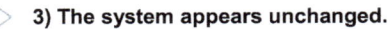 3) The system appears unchanged.

4) The pigs use the external influence to turn to the food.

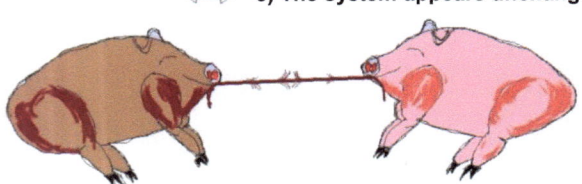

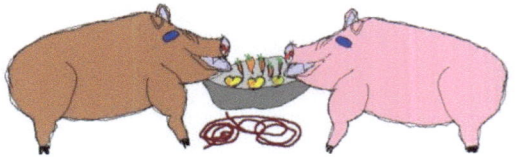

A system can also 'neutralise' external influences. The ability to maintain a state independently is characteristic of living systems (e.g. plants).

Or a system may show up something 'surprising'. Only animals and people have the ability to act independently from any external influence ('character'). In addition, only humans are able to shape their own character and resonate actively with spirituality.

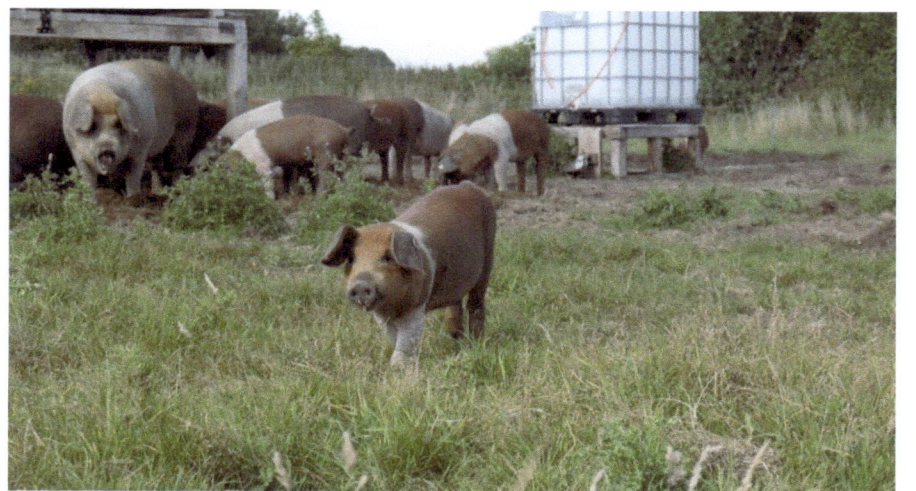
(NF)

Calm - making decisions - doing - step by step - that's all pig!

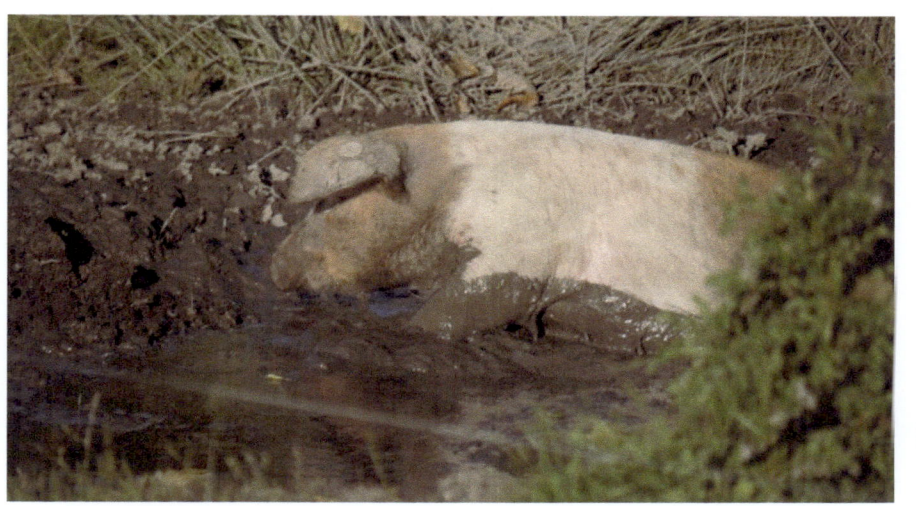
(NF)

Everything that is able to give or receive joy needs special attention and protection.

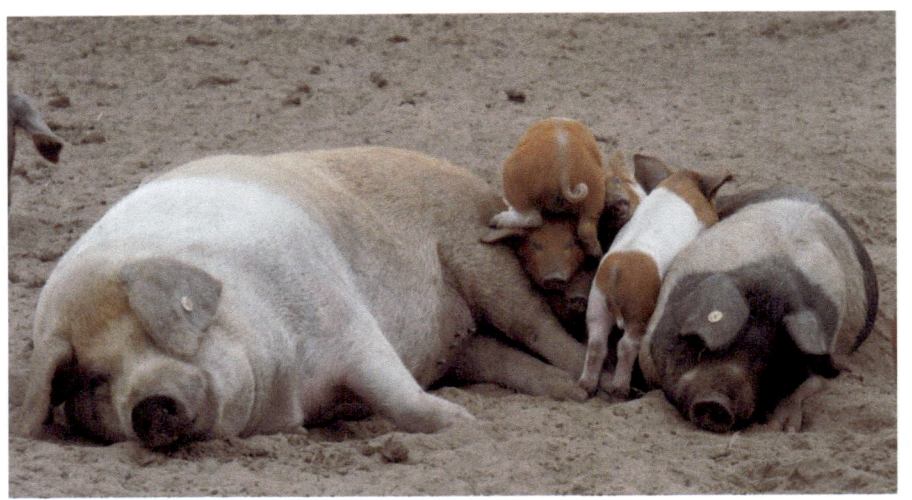

(NF)

Physical acts of (Christian) mercy are: feeding the hungry, taking in the homeless, clothing the naked, visiting the sick and those in prisons, burying the dead, giving alms (which is also one of the five pillars of Islam. In today's society: unconditional basic income?)

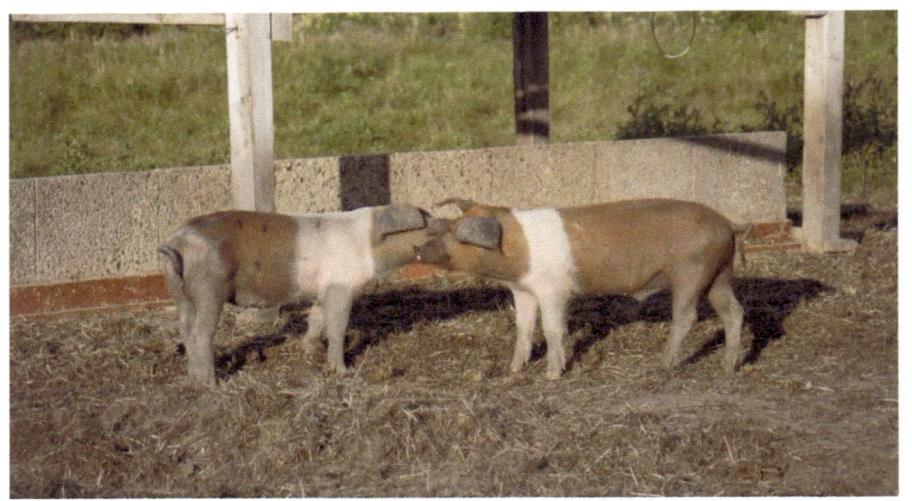

(NF)

Spiritual acts of (Christian) mercy are: teaching the ignorant, advising the doubting, comforting the grieving, admonishing the sinner, freely forgiving the bully, patiently tolerating the annoying, praying for the living and the dead.

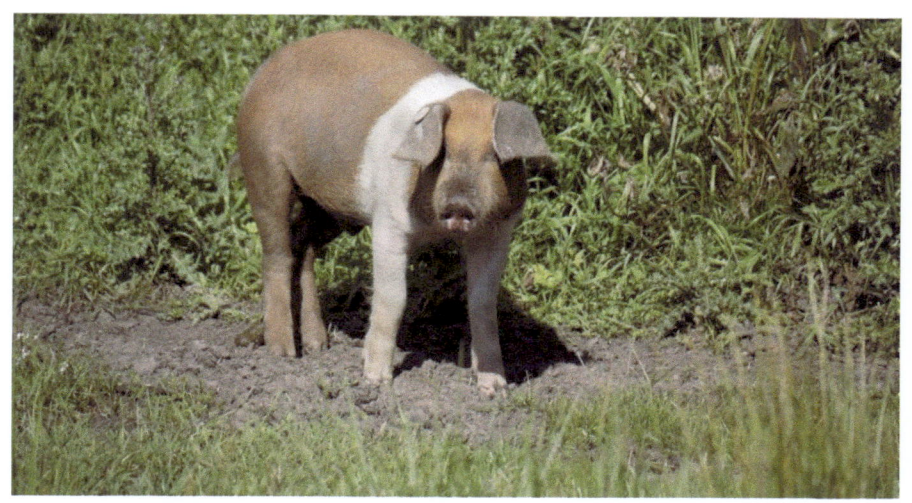
(NF)

In Buddhism these actions and qualities are considered as liberating: generosity, meaningful actions, patience, joyful effort, meditation, wisdom, love, empathy, sharing others' joy, equilibrium.
Islamic virtues are: humility, refraining from thoughtless and superficial talk, payment of 'zakat' (a religious alms tax), modesty, taking care of goods and tasks which have been entrusted to you, prayer ('salat').

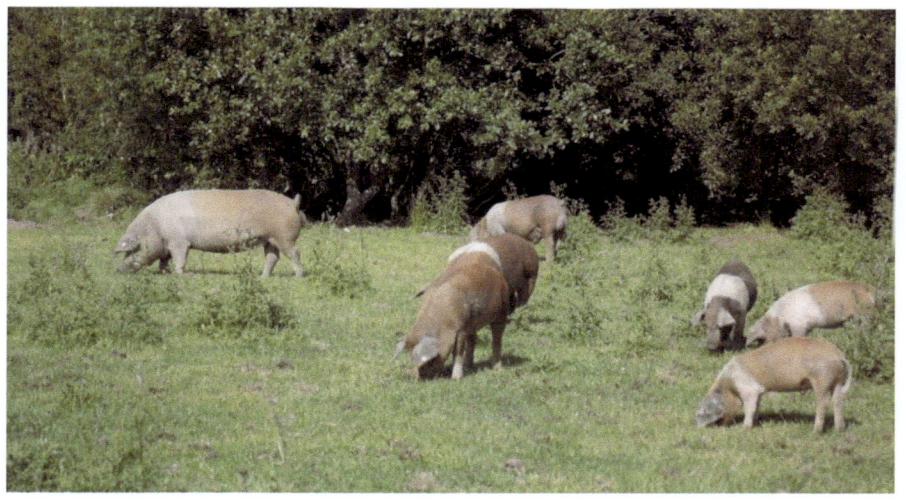
(NF)

In a nutshell: we need to live in a way which we regard as the right way, in both word and deed, and hope that our vibrations will resonate with others.

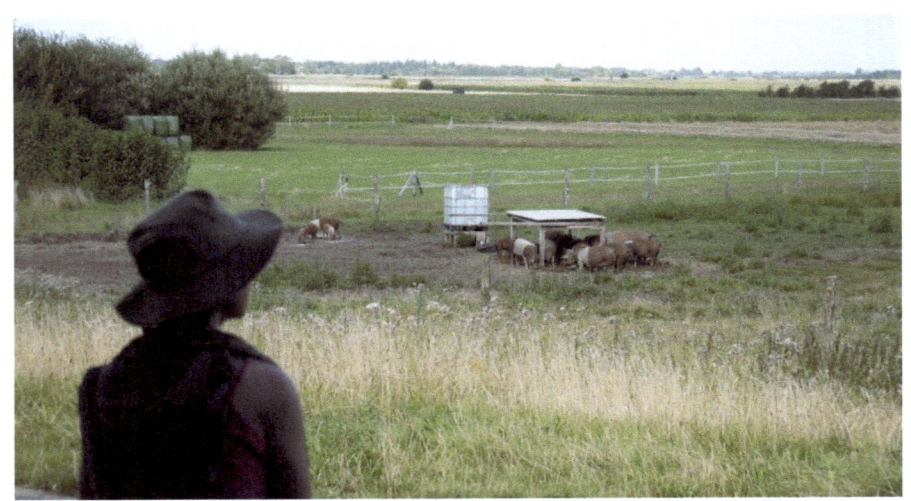
(NF)

Be it pigs, music, nature, adventure, sport, culture or people - Our spiritual 'Ego' will reach us as part of our opening up to and resonating with our spirituality - in the form of joy, an inner voice, intuitive knowledge, inner certainty (belief), a guardian angel. ("Joy, beautiful spark of the divinity..." ("*Freude, schöner Götterfunken...*" [Schiller])),
Such belief 'happens' it cannot be demanded.

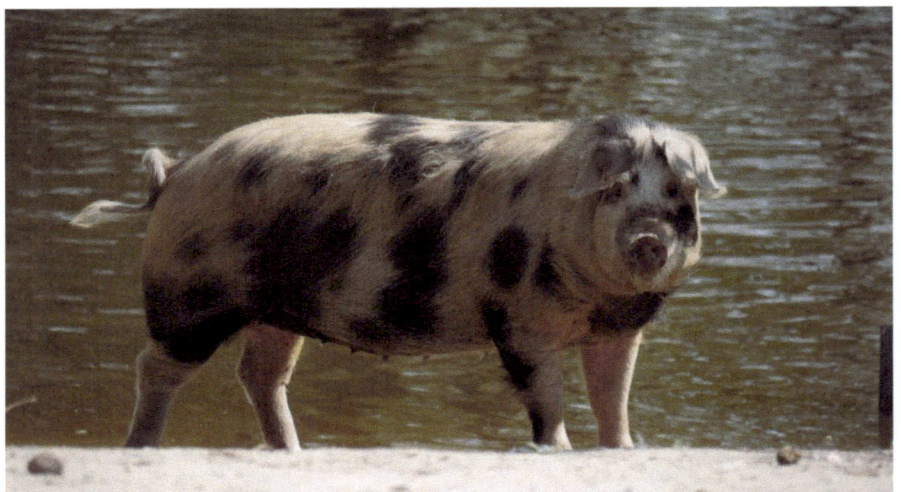
(RD)

We may choose to lie to others, but lying to ourselves will not do us any favours. Gnothi seauton – know yourself (inscription at the Apollo Temple in Delphi // We only know what we believe.// "Sincerity is the best medicine against lack of self-confidence" [Tenzin Gyatso, 14. Dalai Lama]

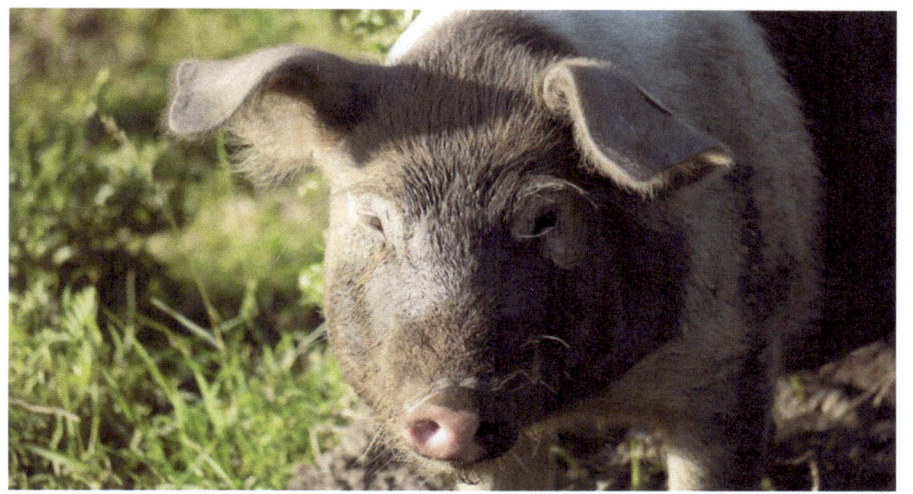
(NF)

Those who are not acutely aware of the stirrings of their soul are inevitably unhappy. [Marc Aurel]

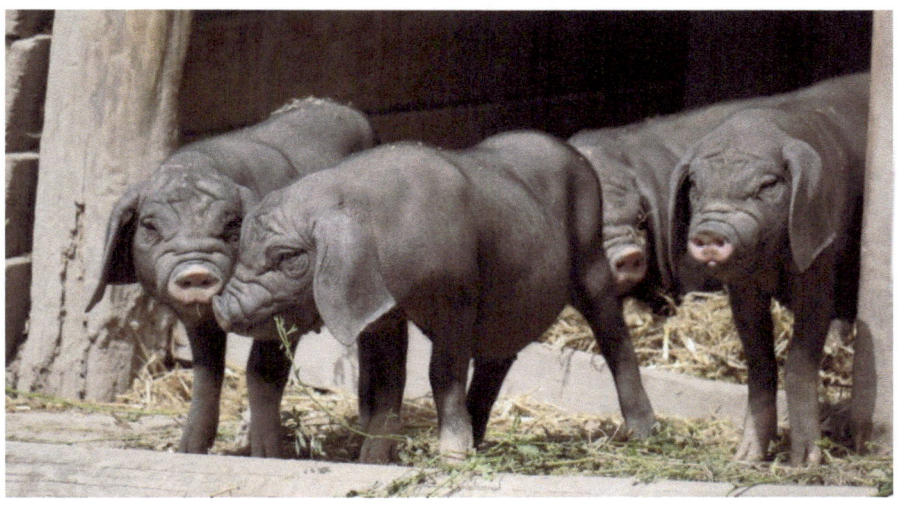
(LRO)

Protection from arbitrariness is the responsibility of the individual - much to the frustration of those obsessed with order.

In conclusion

What has this booklet given us?
Maybe some thoughts for our future paths... as well as - we hope - sheer delight in all those cute piglets.
- That the indivudal is responsible for their aspirations. In particular, an individual is accountable for their intention and care taken, the perspective they choose and the effort they give to understanding, more so than the specific outcome of any particular act.
- That spirituality is an option for better understanding of oneself and of others.
- That the existence of an independent universal spirituality does not contradict today's scientific world view, but seems rather comparable to the relationship between imaginary numbers and natural numbers. (and who would have expected that we can 'prove' 'i' [$i^2 =-1$] using natural numbers?) Nowadays a comparison with the virtual worlds of Internet and clouds may well be more accessible.
- When making decisions: That knowledge gained from spiritual insight may be just as valuable as 'gut feeling', the opinion of others and rational analysis. That decisions made in harmony with our beliefs free us of feelings of guilt, yet remain open to change.
- That there is no human or factual justification to question another's certainties, as long as they are not mere convictions or generalisations.
- That the harmonious resonance with our individual spiritual pattern is experienced as joy.
- That we concede the opportunity to experience joy to all people (and sensitive creatures).

When I gathered the pictures and texts for this booklet I 'accidentally' came across Bronnie Ware's fascinating book: The Top Five Regrets of the Dying. While I have some reservations about her book, her experiences and messages are relevant for anyone wishing to make life changing decisions:
Top regret of the dying is not to have had the courage to live his or her own life. And wishing they had allowed themselves more joy. According to Ware, many people realise only at the end of their lives that happiness and joy are choices we can make.
With this booklet I hope to have offered an impulse for courage and responsibility for our life joy.

Gudrun Bornhöft   Goslar, November 2016

And here is another thought to conclude:
What if everything is already in place and we merely travel through the (spiritual) landscape as if on a train?
Just a thought!

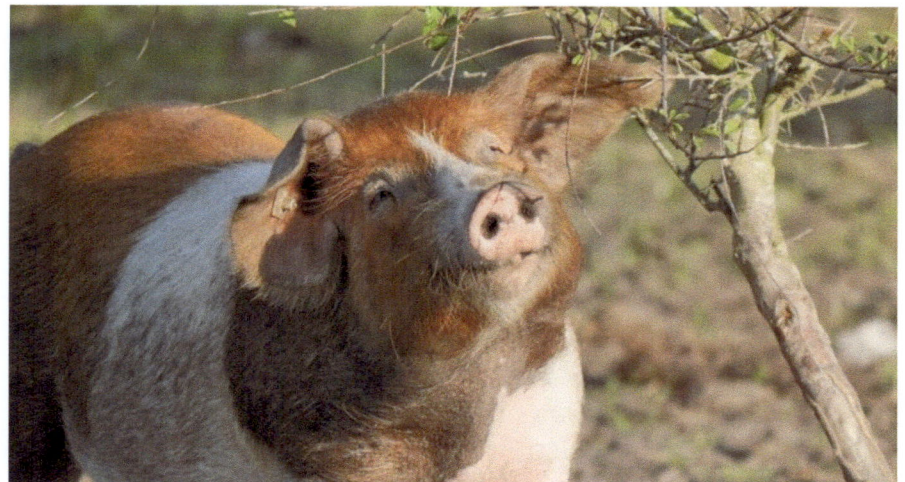

(NF)

"But the fruit of the Spirit is love, joy, peace, forbearance, kindness, goodness, faithfulness, gentleness and self-control.......Since we live by the Spirit, let us keep in step with the Spirit." [Gal 5,22...5,25}

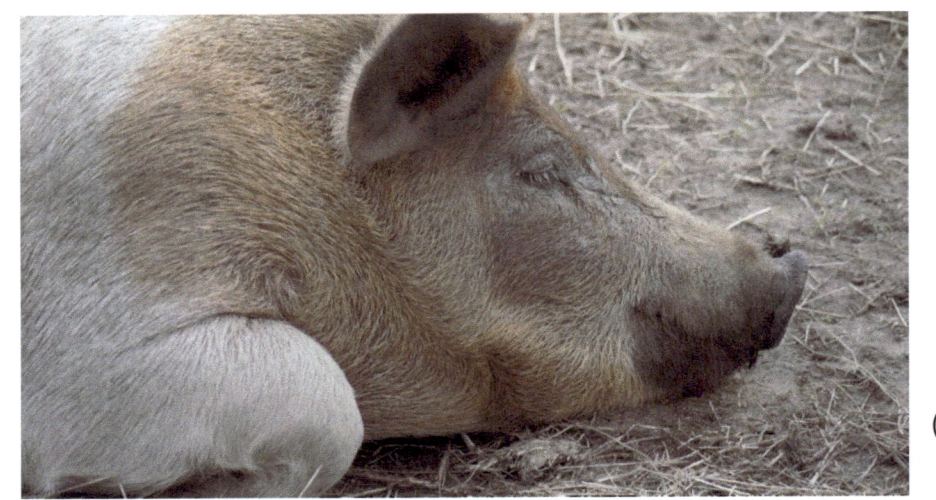 (NF)

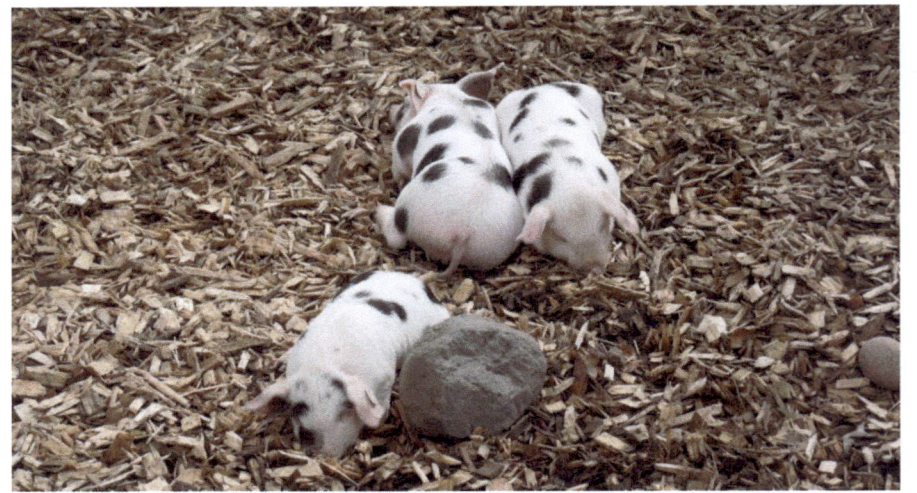 (RD)